Lose the Sugar,
You're Sweet Enough

Karen Calandra

Registered Nurse

Certified Holistic Health Coach

Copyright

This book is a guide that uses Whole Food as Prescription to Better Health. Everybody is different, so if you have any unique or special medical conditions, dietary restrictions, food allergies, pregnant, nursing, diabetic, or on anticoagulation therapy please consult your physician promptly before attempting this detoxification and eating plan. This book is to be used for informational purposes and is not to replace or be a substitute for the advice of your personal qualified medical professional, who should always be consulted before beginning any new exercise, nutritional or health plan.

All efforts have been made to ensure that the information herein is accurate and up to date. The author assumes no responsibility for any adverse effects arising from the use or application of the information contained herein.

Dedication

To my One and Only God, Thank you for having a GREAT plan for my life. I have found gratification and passion in being blessed to share my talents and gifts with so many as I help and nurture your beautiful children to respect the one and only temple you have gifted them with. It is truly an Honor to guide them along their special journey to be "The Best They Can Be."

To my amazing husband, my best friend, my partner in life, Sal, who allows me to be myself and pursue my passions with enthusiasm and support. Thank you for always being there for me and loving me so much. I will love you forever and it's true I do love you more!

To my dear and loving children, Joshua, Salvatore and Michael and my granddaughter Skylar Tate. I adore and love you more than words can express. It is my hope that the guidelines in this book will help you all be healthier and adopt life-styles, as you grow older to be healthier and happier in the years to come.

To my niece, Katie, thank you for all the hours and professionalism spent doing my cover. It was fun collaborating with you. I absolutely love it!

To my mentor, Robbie Raugh R.N. You have taught me a great deal and I love that we are partners in helping change this health care crisis one person at a time. Together we are part of the ripple effect and we are strong!

My editors, Zendi Moldenhauer PhD, NPP, PNP, RN-BC and Joell Stephens, I appreciate all the time you spent editing, advising and for being so patient with me.

To the Institute of Integrated Nutrition, thank you for believing in me and opening the doors of opportunity for a better future.

To my parents, my siblings, and extended families, Thank you for all the support and for making even small changes in your diet and lifestyle to better your own health so we can spend many more years together.

I love you all.

Table of Content

Introduction

We live in a crazy world troubled by an epidemic of obesity and sickness; our health care system is focused on sick care. It seems as though money is spent on treating symptoms of disease instead of getting to the root cause. Over the last twenty years, I have seen the devastation of what poor dietary habits have done to so many people including myself. After a recent health scare with thyroid cancer and my own personal journey with psoriatic arthritis, this led me on a quest to heal myself and learn all I could about the food industry and the food I've been consuming. I had been a yo-yo dieter for twenty-two years, name the diet, and I've been on it! I've counted calories, points, and I even went low fat in the eighties and tried restrictive diets thinking I was doing good things for my body. I have come to realize that my sugar filled life in many ways was causing me to be ill. As a nurse, I was taught about the relationship between food and health, but I was never taught about how nutrition affects our health and wellness. Today's food is causing many of us to be sick, and it seems that inflammation is at the heart of many chronic conditions these days. After going back to school to be educated about nutrition, I now understand more and I am still learning everyday about how essential good whole food is to our health. During my training, I studied over 100 dietary theories, practical lifestyle management techniques, and innovative coaching methods with some of the world's top health and wellness experts. My teachers included Dr. Andrew Weil, Director of the Arizona Center for Integrative Medicine; Dr. Deepak Chopra, leader in the field of mind-body medicine; Dr. David Katz, Director of Yale University's Prevention Research Center; Dr. Walter Willett, Chair of Nutrition at Harvard University; Geneen Roth, bestselling author and expert on emotional eating; and many other leading researchers and nutrition authorities.

Through my healing processes, I took control over my own eating habits, and I found a balance between the mind, body and spirit; and I have finally learned the prescription to a better health. I am so excited and honored to be able to share this secret with you. As you look around, you will see young children, teens, and adults sadly overweight in the USA. Do you know why? I'm here to tell you that a diet high in processed food, excessive sugar, and stress are keeping our bodies from healing itself. Have you ever heard of the SAD diet (The Standard American Diet)? Nowadays, most Americans eat fast foods, packaged foods in boxes, bags, or anything quick and easy to prepare, I have learned that these foods are the number one reason most people in our nation are very sick.

Most approaches to nutrition dwell on calories, carbohydrates, fats, and proteins. We've been inundated with phrases like "eat less, exercise more" or "calories in equal calories out." Instead of creating lists of restrictions of good and bad foods, I coach my clients to create a happy, healthy life in a way that is flexible, fun, and free of denial and discipline without deprivation, starvation or guilt. I hope to empower you to become an active participant in your own healing by implementing dietary and lifestyle changes that will not only help you reach your goals but produce long term benefits. I am not claiming to be an expert, but I come from a place where many of you can relate. I've struggled for twenty-two years with my weight. I've been on every diet imaginable, and whenever I would put all that weight back on and then some I would feel like a failure. Since then, I've learned that diets do not work; diets are what failed me. There was a struggle with food that raged inside of me, and for many years I made it all about my clothing size or that number on the scale, but it ends up that I really needed to yield to my higher power to get the strength I needed to stop with the foods I thought were giving me comfort. Foods cannot comfort you, and certain foods can be harming you, without you even knowing it. The wonderful news is, I have knowledge and experience that by making healthy choices and eating good whole foods from the earth that those very foods can heal us. Throughout my journey, I found the perfect prescription to better health, and who knew that by eating just good whole foods from the earth that it would be the best prescription, and only prescription to good vibrant health! My excuses have stopped, and I am no longer food deprived. Through changing my diet and incorporating a healthier life-style I have lost 30 pounds and I have kept it off. Not only have I, lost more weight in a 12-week period of time than ever before but my psoriasis has cleared, my psoriatic arthritis is much better, I have more energy than ever before and I even sleep better. I could go on and on about the benefits of good whole natural foods and how my body has responded miraculously, but instead I would like to share it with you. You may be thinking, will it work for you? Indeed it will!

Is it that easy? Yes, it is! However, you must be ready to stop the sugar madness? Are you willing to stop with the excuses and start today? If you are, we can begin your journey today to better health. The sugar in our processed food has taken over our taste buds. We need to lose the sugar, friends. This prescription just may save your life!

It's time to stop the nonsense and get serious, and take matters into your own hands. Be proactive and start making better choices with the food you eat. The idea is not to wait until you have a disease; the idea is to start now so disease doesn't have the chance to develop, but do not fret if you already have a disease because some diseases, may be reversed, so it is not too late to start following this prescription to better health. You will slowly begin to transform, and all your previous struggles may become a thing of the past.

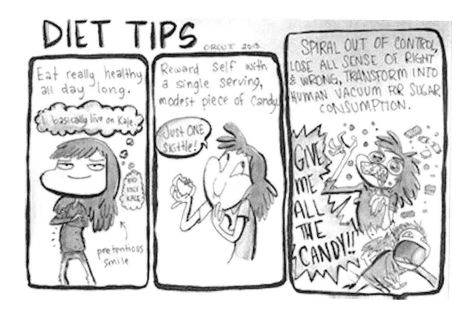

Chapter 1

Lose the Sugar, Not the Fat

Did you know fat is not making us fat? In the 1980s it was decided that fat was the main cause of heart disease so manufacturers began making low fat products and nonfat items in hopes to reduce heart disease. However, to keep food tasting good they replaced the fat with sugar. Sugar is now what is making us fat, sugar is the main reason we have an epidemic of obesity. According to the Department of Health and Human Services, the truth is that during the last 20 years the percentage of young people who are obese has tripled. Hospital costs have increased to 31 billion dollars for cardiovascular disease related to obesity. Doctors agree the more overweight a person is the more likely he or she is to have health problems. Excess sugar causes inflammation in our bodies, which is putting our bodies at a huge health care risk. I believe, sugar is the cause of obesity, and obesity raises the risk of many health conditions: high blood pressure, stroke, diabetes, heart disease, gall bladder, infertility, osteoarthritis, respiratory problems, sleep apnea, colon, breast and endometrial cancers and more. It's time to do something about this now; it's time to take control over what we are putting into our mouths. Would you eat 22 packs of sugar? Well, if you drink a can of soda, you just consumed 22 packs of sugar. Dr. Mark Hyman says, "The average American eats 152 pounds of sugar in one year." That's over one pound for every man, woman, and child per day. Sugar triggers overeating; it's a physiological response because your body demands it. Sugar is truly an addiction and even more addictive than cocaine. If you are currently eating foods high in sugar and processed foods in your diet, you are addicted to sugar. Many do not realize the dangers of sugar, all you know is that it tastes good and you want more. The addiction to sugar and simple carbohydrates causes insulin imbalance and stores fat in our bodies. Sugar spikes our insulin and causes inflammation, both of which eventually lead to disease. The time is now folks. We have to stop the sugar madness! We must lose the sugar in our diets and learn to eat low glycemic to keep disease at bay and do our best to reverse disease if you already have it.

How might you do this, you may ask? Well, the first thing is to reduce the sugar, flour, and processed food in our diet. My suggestion is a detoxification. Nowadays, there are many detoxifications, but I'm talking about incorporating just good whole natural foods from the Earth; it's time to ditch the sugar: it's the only way! Detoxifying is not deprivation; it is about eating an abundance of good whole natural foods. The body can heal itself by taking out some of the processed foods and adding good healthy whole foods. You can eat as many vegetables as you want. You will not get fat eating good whole vegetables from the Earth!

Why should you detoxify? Whenever beginning a healthy transformation for your body, it's helpful to begin by cleansing your body with a detoxification. It's important to cleanse your system of harmful toxins. The pesticides, herbicides, and fungicides that are sprayed on our fruits and vegetables are some of the many toxins that need to be eliminated from your body. In addition, there are many chemicals, natural flavorings, dyes, fast foods, fat, trans-fat, sugar-laden foods, antibiotics, hormones, caffeine, alcohol, and refined vegetable oils that have dirtied our internal filters. Even the air we breathe and water we drink have pollutants. Our internal systems are loaded with environmental and external toxins. All these toxins puts poison in our bodies, and those toxins can cause chronic diseases, autoimmune problems, degenerative diseases, allergies, neurological and digestive disorders, cardiovascular diseases, hormone imbalances, obesity, cancers and more! I know it's difficult to control everything in our environment, but one thing we have control over is what we put into our mouths.

To maintain good health or regain good health, detoxifying is a GREAT way start. Detoxifying will help to clean up our internal filters to reduce inflammation. Through a detoxifying program it will clean up our liver and our digestive tract, and can feed the body with foods that are easy for the body to digest. Losing the sugar, combined with a three to seven day detoxification, and then followed by a good healthy nutritional lifetime eating plan that includes, good exercise, adequate hydration, supplements, stress reduction, and the proper amount of sleep, I believe is the prescription we all need. If you follow this plan, you will have the perfect prescription to a healthy long life hopefully without illness. I know that's my goal, how about you?

Chapter 2

Detoxification and Journaling

The detoxification is simple, and it is a healing prescription for everyone. There is nothing scary about eating just vegetables and fruit. Plant based foods are actually safe to eat, and the detoxification process should last three to seven days. I encourage the full seven days if you can challenge yourself to do it. You can do anything for a week right? Although it will be a huge change to the way you are currently eating, I promise you it will be worth it! It may seem like the longest week in your life, and it may not be easy but it will set you up not only to have success through the program but also to have success for a lifetime. During this program, you will lose fat, inches, and notice your clothes fitting better while building muscle. Do not weigh yourself every day because the weight did not come on in a day, so you will not lose it all in a day. Be patient and kind to yourself.

To start, you need the following tools to help you become successful in your new journey to a healthier life: a scale, tape measure, a journal to record in, and the ability to go shopping for your vegetables and fruit. The next thing you need to do is record your measurements and monitor your results every month so you can see progress; measure the circumference of your chest, waist, hips, and thighs with a tape measure and record it into a journal along with your weight without shoes.

Record your current activity level and be honest with this assessment, you may even want to take a before and after photo. The results will motivate you and you will feel more empowered by the experience.

The following foods that are not permitted during detoxification week: white potatoes, white rice, white bread, or any grains (to check for gluten and or glyphosate intolerances or sensitivities), fats, oils, alcohol, coffee, soda or other caffeine drinks, sugar, artificial sweeteners, dairy, junk food, beans, nuts or seeds. Dairy, nuts or seeds are not permitted during the detoxification because they contain fat and fat takes longer to digest. Fats, whether good or bad, are still fats, and if you're trying to detoxify your system you need to eliminate them during this time. That's why even raw nuts, organic milk, and organic eggs are not recommended during the detoxification week. Organic dairy is acidic and mucous forming. The goal is to try to alkalinize your body to lower or minimize inflammation. Inflammation is the precursor to all disease. You can use vegan plant based hemp shakes with water during detox.

For the Detoxification, it's important to eat a rainbow of vegetables. You can eat as many vegetables as you'd like and be sure to get in greens on a daily basis. Spinach and kale are great protein sources so be sure to have a salad at least once a day but preferably twice a day.

Many people always ask, "Don't I need carbohydrates for energy?"

Indeed you do. Did you know that vegetables are complex carbohydrates? Carbohydrates are made from molecules of sugar, and when they are found in vegetables, nuts, and seeds, they are called complex carbohydrates. Complex carbohydrates will help you feel fuller longer because they take longer to break down and digest better because and they have the added fiber you need. This energy is released slower than simple carbohydrates, which release energy quicker, and dumps a lot more sugar into the bloodstream. The simple carbohydrates are without fiber and are filled with empty calories. We need to eliminate all simple, man-made, processed carbohydrates to keep our blood sugar at an even level. Simple carbohydrates to eliminate: breads, pastries, sweets, fruit juices or anything in a box, bag or carton that lack fiber, fat, and protein. Eliminating these foods will keep our bodies' low glycemic and low in SUGAR. To understand low glycemic one needs to understand the way carbohydrates affect out blood sugar. All carbohydrates are not equal. We should eat vegetable carbohydrates that are high in fiber; fat and protein. After detoxification, you may add beans, nuts, and steel cut oats. They help us to stay fuller longer and they digest slower. However, during detoxification you can eat as many vegetables as you would like. As a matter of fact, you should eat vegetables at any time for the rest of your life! The only vegetables you are not permitted to eat are the sweet potatoes, winter squash, and beets but just during the 3 to 7 days of detoxification. Remember raw is always preferred, but you can roast, steam, grill or sauté them in some vegetable or chicken broth. Feel free to juice your vegetables in a juicer along with eating them during this week if you prefer.

Detoxifying with good whole fruits and vegetables is the BEST way to start!

You do not need to do shakes, bars or buy special food. Shopping will be simplified as you buy just fruits and vegetables, organic herbal decaffeinated teas and water. Eat them anyway you prefer. Choose a variety and be sure you are getting all the colors of the rainbow. Buying organic from the following list is preferred the fewer chemicals you put into your body the better protection you have against disease.

Here is a list below of the "dirty dozen" which are the most contaminated of vegetables and fruit according to the EWG. You can refer to the Environmental Working Group for the (EWG's) 2014 Shoppers Guide to Pesticides in Produce.

Dirty Dozen-List
Organic: Apples are the most contaminated and are listed first.
1. Apples
2. Strawberries and blueberries
3. Celery
4. Cherry tomatoes and tomatoes
5. Cucumbers
6. Grapes
7. Hot peppers

8. Nectarines
9. Peaches
10. Bell peppers
11. Kale/collard greens and spinach
12. White Potatoes

The clean 15 that do NOT have to be organic are below. Clean means that it has only 1% of pesticide residue on it. Avocados are the cleanest, which is why they are listed first.
1. Avocado
2. Asparagus
3. Cabbage
4. Cantaloupe
5. Eggplant
6. Grapefruit
7. Kiwi
8. Mangos
9. Mushrooms
10. Onions
11. Papayas
12. Pineapples
13. Sweet peas
14. Bananas
15. Sweet corn

The health benefits of organic foods reduce our risk of exposure to unwanted chemicals in your body. This is a way to get the full effect of the antioxidants and enzymes and phytonutrients to clean our internal systems and protect our bodies from disease. Antioxidants are necessary for disease prevention because studies show that they combat free radicals that can cause disease. Free radicals do our bodies harm as they cause inflammation that can lead to infections, heart disease, and some cancers that can affect and impair our immune systems. Fresh fruits and vegetables contain living enzymes that help break down the food in our gastrointestinal tract which supports rest, repair, and rejuvenation. Just detoxifying for 3 to 7 full days will make you feel like a brand new person, and you will have more energy, less joint discomfort, your tummy will feel flatter, and you will find that you will be sleeping better. A detox will set you up for success for the rest of the program. Detoxing jump-starts your weight loss and cleanses your taste buds, your GI tract and your liver. Raw is best unless you have underlying Crohn's disease (please consult your physician if you have intestinal disease) but you can roast, steam or sauté vegetables as well. You can eat as many vegetables as you would like. Each day, I encourage a minimum of 3-5 cups per meal 3 times a day. That is between 9 and 15 cups of vegetables a day! How much are you currently eating? Fruit is another story. You can have 3 fruits the first week. The reason limited fruit is important is because fruit contains a high amount of fructose, and although it digests more slowly than pure glucose, it still stimulates the pancreas to secrete insulin. After your glycogen stores get filled, let's say the tank is full, extra glucose in our body is converted into fat by the liver and is stored as adipose tissue (body fat) in places we prefer it not be stored, like the butt, thighs or our waist. So during the week long detoxification process only three medium size fruits are recommended per day. The benefits of fresh whole fruits are that they provide you with the minerals, nutrients and fiber and they are lower in calories. During your detoxification week you may want to make a detox soups.

VEGETABLE DETOX SOUP

1 carton of organic low sodium chicken broth 1 carton of organic vegetable broth
1 cup of carrots
1 cup of green beans
1 cup of celery
1 cup of onions
1 bag of shredded cabbage (prefer white not purple cabbage as it makes a purple soup)
1 cup of zucchini
2-3 cut up tomatoes
Any spices you like garlic, basil, oregano or "Spike" which is a combination of herbs and spices. Cook until vegetables are tender, approximately 20-30 minutes.

CARROT LEEK SOUP

1 carton of organic vegetable broth
1 carton of organic chicken broth
One bunch of leeks (cleaned and sliced)
One bag of carrots (cleaned and sliced)
And spices of choice, cook for 20-30 minutes until carrots are tender.
These soups are your go to foods. You can eat it for a snack, have it for breakfast or a meal.

Another important process during your detoxification is water. Filtered water is a necessity! The benefits of water include flushing out toxins from your organs, carrying nutrients to all cells, and keeping your body hydrated. Water makes up 60% of your body weight. There are no standard recommendations for the amount of water to drink per day because everyone's body type is different and so is their activity levels. For this program, it is recommended to drink at least one, 8oz. glass of water with lemon half-hour before you even have breakfast to help activate the digestive tract. Water with lemon helps to prepare your stomach and get the gastric juices flowing for the day. Also, try to drink one glass of water before all meals to help improve digestion and fill you up a bit before adding food to your stomach. Be careful if you have low stomach acid production, the water may dilute your stomach acids. If that's the case you may benefit from adding a digestive enzyme before your meal. The general recommendations are about 13 cups for men and 9 cups for women for the day or if it is easier to remember eight, 8oz. glasses of fluid a day. This is just an estimate some may require more.

Journaling is another important component to this perfect prescription to a better life. I highly encourage journaling because it will help you better understand what food allergies you may have along with what food makes you feel great. Also, journaling your food may be helpful to assess the amount of food intake, to be sure you are eating enough and drinking the recommended amount of water. Writing down your feelings is as equally as important to writing down what you eat: write the good, the bad, and the ugly. Expressing your feelings on paper may help you identify and change unhealthy patterns. It is important to identify why you feel as you do and to see if you are an emotional eater. Most of us are! We eat for happy occasions, sad occasions, when we're angry, feeling stressed, or out of complete boredom. It is the way we are. Food has been associated with feelings of comfort and pleasure. It can also make us feel shameful and can be addicting. We need to recognize what category we fall into, so we can identify and make the appropriate changes. These feelings will not help you accomplish your goals unless you address them and work through them so you not only will have physical growth but good mental health as well. They both work together for optimal wellness and healing. The research shows that when people write down everything that they put into their mouth, they have more success than those who do not and who pretend certain things don't enter their mouths. You understand where I'm going with this, right? Besides writing down every food that enters your mouth, it's important to write your feelings because that's the only way you change the course of action in the future. When you're stressed and looking for food, write that down in your journal. The reason for this is and many of you may be able to relate to this scenario, when you reflect back into the journal when you've had a bad day and you ate a carton of ice cream before dinner, got mad at yourself and vowed to never let it happen again. By writing that all down helps you to recognize it the next time and will allow you to change the action! Instead of eating a bag of chips or ice cream you may now make a conscious decision to go for a walk or clean a closet or have some soup instead! It's necessary to recognize the relationship we have with our emotions and food and find ways to replace unhealthy foods. Journaling helps us to be aware and cognizant of our feelings allowing us to find the alternatives. Similarly, let's say you're eating broccoli, wheat, or dairy and it's not agreeing with you. If you are writing down how you feel daily and you are bloated or gassy after eating a certain food, then you may have an intolerance or sensitivity to that food. If that is the case you may not want to put that food into your body as often. What is okay for one person to eat may be like a poison to the next, so you see, journaling is very important.

Another example is perhaps you reach a plateau and you see no weight loss or loss of inches in a four-week period. You can then look back in your journal and most likely find out why. Maybe it means you're eating the wrong foods too frequently, or maybe you need to bump the intensity of your workout or increase the amount of days you go to the gym. Either way you will realize what you need to change if all is written down in your journal, so you can look back to reflect. The biggest challenge here is changing the way we think about our relationship emotionally to food and finding healthier options.

Journaling helps tell the truth about what's really going on in your life and in your body and helps you explore how your mind and body responds to different foods. So buy yourself a notebook, keep it in your purse or on the kitchen counter and write down the foods you eat and how you feel afterwards, do this daily. No one will see it but you, so be honest.

I have to admit that I have realized through my own journaling that I was a stressful eater in the past and that helped me significantly change the way I look at food now. Just because I have lost 30 pounds and have been able to keep it off for years doesn't mean that I still don't go looking for the wrong foods when I am upset or distressed about something. Biggest advantage is that I now recognize those emotions and what I do is find a healthy substitute. When I am stressed and looking for something sweet, I use a tablespoon of natural organic peanut or nut butter and then mix it with a teaspoon of organic fruit spread. It's a whole lot better for me than the sleeve of cookies or slice of chocolate cake I used to eat and it helps me get through that emotional moment when I need something sweet. The fiber protein mix always does the trick! Other times I'll go right to a messy closet or drawer and begin cleaning it out. It takes my mind off the emotion and when I finished the chore I feel accomplished. You will find your own healthier options if you recognize the times when you are stressed.

Since I'm talking about emotions, I'd like to address the guilty feelings associated with foods. The foods we eat and then beat ourselves up mentally over. Balance is truly the key with this program. If I told you, you could never have another piece of cake again you would probably run so fast the other way, right? Well, so would I. It's important when you reach your weight loss goals to balance your foods with an 80- 20 rule. Eighty percent of the time you eat good whole foods from the earth, Twenty percent of the time you indulge in some food that may not be the healthiest for you but foods you enjoy eating. Those foods could be a cultural thing or a food that has been in your family for years that you do not want to give up completely. Do NOT feel guilty when you indulge or when you are not eating perfectly every meal or snack. Do not punish yourself when you've been away on a vacation and enjoyed foods that you do not normally eat. These are the times when you get back on the horse after a vacation, go through a 3-7 day detox and cleanse your body. I believe this to be a healthy balance that will keep our bodies less inflamed and help decrease disease. That is the ultimate goal here. Decreasing our risk for disease by eating good whole foods. What most fail to realize is ninety-eight percent of eating healthy is mental. We get to decide what goes into our mouths. We are the ones responsible for our choices, no one forces us. So by making good healthy choices 80% of the time and indulging 20% on not so great choices keeps a healthy balance and allows you to not feel deprivation. It's all a state of mind.

Preparation is the key to keeping you on track and your success. It's important to shop and prepare your vegetables weekly. Please do not go shopping hungry. If you have everything ready for each meal ahead of time you have a plan. Cook once and eat twice or three times, last night's dinner can become tomorrow's lunch, freezing leftovers for another time. Make hard-boiled eggs for protein after the detox and always keep them on hand. Start using your Crockpot and a Vitamix for soups. Plan your meals for the week and make a grocery list to make shopping easy and less stressful. A plan will help you with success and keep you from making impulsive unhealthy and unwanted choices. The beginning organization is hard because it is helping you develop a new habit of planning and shopping, but once you start doing this it becomes second nature and you won't even need to put much thought into it.

Salads are great for lunch, but for now, during the detoxification ditch the dressing or you can make one with water or vinegar, but no oil. I like to make salads for the week in mason jars with the wide mouths. Dressing always goes first then put in tomatoes, carrots, celery, onions, cucumbers, and top with spinach, arugula or kale or mixed leafy greens. Fill to the top so there is no air left in the jars and they will stay fresh for one full week.

Here is a simple detox dressing to use:

One half cup of Bragg's Apple Cider Vinegar
Salt and Pepper to taste
1-2 teaspoons stone ground mustard
2 teaspoons of any fresh herb: cilantro, parsley, and basil
Whisk all ingredients

Feel free to juice vegetables or add green drinks. It's a great way to add kale, spinach, cucumbers, and other vegetables to get the necessary vitamins and minerals for a healthier diet. There are many clean eating websites and books on juicing and green smoothies. I do suggest you invest in a NutriBullet or a Vitamix for smoothies or a Breville Juicer for juicing. I have all three of these brands and like them very much. To prepare you must: shop, clean and cut up veggies, place in zip lock bags or containers and label with the day of the week, so when you leave for work in the morning you have what you need.

Going through a detox isn't an easy week to get through, but I know you can do it! There are some symptoms you may experience during your detoxification week. Many of my clients and I detox approximately four times a year, or after a holiday or vacation, just to clean out toxins that build up in our system over time. This is the lifestyle of which I talk about and live.

If you have been eating a lot of processed sugar and caffeine you may experience a headache on about day three of the detox. Some people may even feel achy and have flu like symptoms; some may have skin breakouts. All this is normal; keep drinking your water to flush out all the nastiness. By day three or four it's possible and likely to begin feeling tired, fatigued and have no energy. There is no vigorous exercising during this week for this very reason, you are not eating any protein and therefore do not want to burn muscle, you need to be kind to yourself, I encourage long walks only. Get some extra rest, relax and don't over exert yourself. This is a good time to start paying attention to how your body feels and respond in kind, but let me tell you by day five you will be starting to feel much better. Day six will bring a renewed sense of energy, thinness around your middle, and possibly a great night sleep. Be patient and start listening to your body. Your hormones will be beginning to change, your taste buds are reestablishing themselves and you are on your way to a lifestyle transformation!

Here is a sample of what a detox day will look like.

First take time to breathe, relax and be grateful for your food. Take time to savor the flavors of the day.

Pre-Breakfast~ One 8 ounce glass of warm water with lemon.

Breakfast~ Plate of vegetables, roasted, sautéed, steamed or raw at least 3 cups or (as much as you would like) and one serving of a medium fruit and one 8 ounce glass of filtered water.

Lunch~ A huge leafy green salad, at least 3 cups with as many vegetables as you would like, and one serving of a medium fruit and one 8oz. glass filtered water.

Snack~ raw veggies (all colors) and vegetable broth or detox soup and one 8 ounce glass of filtered water or organic herbal tea.

Dinner~ A plate of veggies, a salad, soup and one serving of a medium fruit and one 8oz glass of filtered water. Drink water in between meals as well and an organic herbal tea or vegetable broth thought-out the day this will help you stay hydrated, feel full and flush out all the toxins.

Do not skip meals! Even if you are not hungry, to regulate your metabolism your body needs to be fed.

Skipping meals immediately begins fat storage. Do NOT do that to yourself! It is recommended to avoid protein during the detox to get the full detoxification. However, if your body is telling you after three days that you need protein you may add 4 ounce of lean clean, no antibiotic, no hormone chicken, wild fish (tuna or salmon), turkey, tofu, one hard boiled or soft cooked egg or almond milk to either lunch or dinner. You must give the detoxification at least three days, if you haven't given the detoxification three days you may not be ready for this commitment.

If you are a diabetic consult your physician, they may recommend that you detox WITH protein at every meal. Anyone with any special medical problems or dietary needs must consult their physician before attempting these guidelines. Blood sugars drop considerably during the detox week, therefore diabetics on medication will need to be checking in daily with their physician for medication adjustments.

Once you have completed ONE week of detoxification, I guarantee you will feel like a new person. You will be smiling, feeling energized, and so pleased with your accomplishment. I don't even know you personally, but if you're reading this book and completed this detoxification, I'm proud of you! It tells me that you are taking this new journey seriously and you want to make healthier changes in your life. You are on your way to better health I am so excited for you! Making these proactive healthy lifestyle changes shows you care and love yourself. I'm smiling from ear to ear, so congratulations to all of you who have gotten this far. It's the best defense we have right now to decrease our cravings for sugar, keep disease away, reverse disease and be the BEST we can be!

Okay, you made it through the detoxification week. Good for you! I bet you feel GREAT ~finally you are making YOU a priority! Now it's time to understand that "Food is Medicine." Our bodies were designed to heal themselves when we put the proper nutrition into it. Feeling great is just one example of how food can dictate how you feel; there is a strong relationship with food and mood. The old saying, "You are what you eat" and "You crave what you eat" are very true.

Chapter 3

Eat to Nourish Your Body

We need to get rid of all unwanted food in your pantry's and refrigerators. Anything with a long shelf life needs to go, all processed foods need to go, all junk foods need to go. We need to eat to nourish our bodies. You may have heard the saying that we need to eat to live not live to eat! How true that is! Our bodies were not designed to process junk food, chemicals or all the sugar that has been put in our foods by the food industries. We need to nourish our bodies with nutrient dense foods that will decrease our body fat, increase our muscle mass and increase our energy.

Do you often wonder why we crave fats, sugar, and salt? It's crazy how the food industry has intentionally put bad stuff in our food to make us crave certain foods and cause us to over eat. In addition, the FDA allows foods that are not good for us and maybe responsible for causing disease. Recent documentaries provide amazingly scary insights about the food in America and will turn your stomach and make you be a bit more proactive about what you are putting in your body and your family's. Some of my favorite documentaries include: *Processed People*, *Forks Over Knives*, *Genetic Rolette*, and the new film *Fed Up*.

Be wary of GMO products such as: corn, soy, cottonseed, and sugar beets they are all genetically engineered. GMO stands for Genetically Modified Organisms, which are foods that have been genetically altered from their original state. This practice started around 1996 in the United States, the FDA says these foods do not need to be labeled and they are not required to approve them for consumption. Individual companies claim to go through a voluntary safety review process with the FDA before they are put on the market, I am not comforted by that practice, seems to be a conflict of interest in my opinion. Moreover, there is an escalating political disagreement going on right now between labeling advocates and the food industries, there are 85 pending GMO labeling bills in 29 states last I checked. Proposition 37 was an initiated state statue in California that would require labeling of GMO's and disallow the practice of labeling GMO's with the word "natural" in it. I am very interested in the labeling of GMO foods and am equally concerned about the real reason why in 2013 there was a study by a French Research team that linked GMO corn to tumors in rats; I saw the gruesome photos but yet a scientific publisher cited weak evidence supporting the conclusions so it was retracted. My feeling is this, it took many years before the U.S. Surgeon General first released their report in 1964 that there was a link between lung cancer and smoking. The tobacco industry knew of this connection years earlier and buried their own research for decades before they went public. I think it's just a matter of time before these companies admit how dangerous GMO foods really are to our internal organs and in the meantime I think we have a right to know what foods have GMO ingredients or not. Proposition 37 does not say that companies cannot produce GMO food it simply says "LABEL IT" so my advice is to use the above foods in moderation or not at all, look for the non-GMO versions if possible. If round up is injected into the DNA of vegetables and causes an insect belly to burst, I'm not so sure I want to ingest that food but of course I will leave it up to you.

We need to get back to eating good whole foods that were eaten 20 to 30 years ago.

We just need to eat good whole foods from the Earth!

These are called Nutrient dense foods, which our bodies require for sustainable energy. We need good nutrients like vegetables, fruits, proteins, fats, minerals, vitamins, and whole grains to keep our bodies healthy.

Side note: unfortunately, one-third of America is clinically obese right now. Juvenile diabetes is on the rise, something we never had with our children twenty years ago. It's been said that we have an obese nation void of nutrients. Why is that? It is because the processed foods we are consuming have little to no nutrient value. It's all been made in a processing plant not the plant that grows from the ground with nutrients from the Earth.

Energy, how do we obtain our energy? We get energy from the foods we eat, what we drink, how much we exercise, a good night's sleep, and the air we breathe.

Everything we eat is converted into glucose to be used by our cells along with oxygen. Our insulin, which is secreted by the pancreas, is the gateway or acts as a key to let the glucose into our cells. The problem is when people eat too much glucose or too many foods, like simple carbohydrates that turn into glucose; our body stores that sugar and it turns into fat.

Like I said before: We need to keep our bodies low in sugar. That means we need to eat low glycemic to keep our blood sugar levels constant. It's time to BLAST THROUGH the sugar addiction!

How do we do this?

AFTER 3-7 DAYS OF DETOXING

After your 3-7 day detox, you can resume your exercise regime. It's important to continue to eat foods that give you energy and are considered nutrient dense. Examples of foods high in energy or protein that are filled with nutrients are: arugula, dark leafy greens, spinach, kale, and romaine lettuce. These foods are loaded with vitamins and minerals, fiber and protein. You get the most bang for your buck with nutrient dense foods. In addition to vegetables and fruits, be aware that blueberries are the best antioxidants and a great memory booster You can now add in nuts, eggs, organic grass fed lean meats, beans, wild fish, quinoa, water, coconut, herbal tea, unsweetened plain Greek yogurt, unsweetened almond milk or coconut milk, ginger, lentils, legumes and sesame seeds.

Dark chocolate is good for you as well, be sure it's more than 72% cacao. Dark chocolate improves blood flow and increases brain function, so a small square daily is beneficial and is considered a nutrient dense food.

Keep journaling how you feel after consuming these foods to check for food sensitivities.

Vegetables

Serving size can be 3-5 cups at every meal at the very least or as much as you like any time of the day. The more you eat of these the more weight you will lose. Eat any kind of vegetable you enjoy. Please try new vegetables and fruits every week, your taste buds will change and you may find that your palate will enjoy new varieties. Eat them any way you like; raw, steamed, sautéed, roasted.

NO CORN ~most is genetically modified and it is a grain. ALL corn on the cob is GMO unless it is labeled Non-GMO and you can only have this when you have started adding grain.

Fruits

Enjoy all varieties of fresh fruit but stay away from fruit juices. Limit fruit to no more than 2-3 medium size pieces a day. No dried fruit, they are much higher in sugar. Citrus fruits add a super boost of vitamin C, which helps strengthen your immunity and fights off viruses. Bananas are loaded with potassium and B vitamins and keep our blood sugar more stable. Just remember that the green to yellow bananas are lower on the glycemic index than one with brown spots. All fruits that are over ripen is higher on the glycemic index.

Protein Sources

Protein - a serving size is no larger than your palm, which is approximately 4 ounces for a woman or 6 ounces for a man.

1.) Lean meats, like chicken, hen, turkey without skin, veal, beef, pork, lamb, are allowed for those who are not vegetarians. Organic, no hormone, no antibiotic, free- range grass fed are preferred.

2.) Wild fish not farmed fish is a good source of Omega III to keep our heart healthy and encourage circulation, Salmon, Albacore Tuna, sardines, trout and mackerel are good sources but no more than twice a week for each because of the mercury.

3.) Seafood, shrimp, clams, lobster, calamari, muscles, etc., without butter sauce or fried.

4.) Organic eggs are the perfect protein source, yolk included, and one serving is 1or 2 eggs. Cook them however you prefer and keep hard-boiled eggs on hand to use as a snack or on a salad as a protein source.

5.) Dairy: One cup is the portion for milk. Cow's milk is not recommended unless it's organic due to the hormones and antibiotics. A great alternative is unsweetened almond milk, organic soy, organic rice milk or coconut milk. Organic unsweetened plain Greek yogurt can be eaten and used in smoothies with little fruit and spinach. Please do not buy the yogurt with fruit and sugar additives because the sugar content is too high. Check the ingredient label to be sure the sugar content is no higher than 9 grams per-serving. Organic cheese is also preferred, but limit this to one serving a day of no more than 1-2 ounces.

It's important when eating this way to always be thinking about protein and fiber at every meal. Eat 3-5 cups of vegetables at every meal (three times a day) and add a protein source to it. Two times a day, add a low Glycemic food from the low glycemic list, and eat healthy snacks of fresh fruits or veggies, with hummus.

Caffeine has many pros and cons. A cup of Java in the morning is a liquid pick me up for many. It can increase memory so if you must have one cup a day that's acceptable, but if you can switch to decaffeinated coffee, now is the time. Too much caffeine isn't good for you. Caffeine is a like a drug. We shouldn't be drinking it all day, anything more than 2 cups is not encouraged.

6.) Veggie Garden Burgers are fine just read labels and stay away from ingredients you cannot pronounce. Look for flavorful nutritious organic whole food ingredients. I've heard it said if you cannot pronounce it do NOT eat it.

7.) Tofu-1 cup is a serving of protein.

8.) Nuts & Seeds (One ounce) of all kinds are packed with protein and great sources of minerals but pay attention to the size of a serving. Nine almonds is ONE serving. Too many nuts despite being a good fat will put weight on the hips so be aware. If you do not have a tree nut allergy, enjoy a serving of nuts as a snack or add them to your daily salad. I like to buy slivered almonds or chopped walnuts, tricks me into thinking I'm getting more.

9.) Ground flaxseed- Remember to grind your flaxseed so it's easier for your body to digest. Whole flaxseed may pass through your intestines undigested thereby not receiving the full benefits. One tablespoon of flaxseed contains Omega III, and fiber with little calories. It can lower cholesterol, reduce cardiovascular disease; help with constipation by improving digestive health. Refrigerate to maintain freshness. Like other fiber be sure to drink plenty of fluids such as water. Do not take flaxseed with other medications or supplements but add to cereals, mustard, yogurt, smoothies, muffins or homemade breads. Maximum dosage: 1-tablespoon a day.

Fats

Remember, fat is not making us fat the sugar is! We need good fat! You can begin to add these good fats sparingly. Use a spritzer for oils and remember your serving sizes for meat and nuts. Good fat helps our cardiovascular system and is necessary for cell membrane repair, helps with our hormones, lowers cholesterol, is an antiviral agent and can help protect against cancer. Fats help the body absorb vitamins. Some healthy fats from plants and animals include: olives, olive oil, organic nut oils, coconuts and organic coconut oil unrefined cold pressed, organic butter, avocados, organic eggs, palm oil, grass fed meats, and raw nuts like walnuts and almonds.

Coconut Oil

Organic coconut oil is now called "super food". These fatty acids have amazing capabilities to decrease fat and help our brains function better. It's one of the richest sources of saturated fat that metabolizes by heading straight to the liver and is used as quick energy. The therapeutic effects of coconut help boost brain function, protect skin and hair, improves cholesterol, controls hunger, and decreases infections. It's one of the better fats just be sure to use portion control, 4.5 grams of total fat is in one teaspoon. I use this in place of my butter when making eggs in the morning or add to my smoothies.

Minerals and Vitamins

Minerals and Vitamins perform hundreds of roles in our body. They're considered micronutrients because our body only requires tiny amounts of them for cellular healing, repair, strengthen bones, boost our immune systems, and convert food into energy. They can help eliminate diseases caused by scurvy, rickets, blindness, and prevent birth defects. The major difference between vitamins and minerals is that vitamins can be broken down by heat, air or acid and are more fragile than minerals. Minerals come to us by means of the soil, plants, fish, animals and fluid and hang onto their chemical structure. We cannot manufacture them on our own so it's vitally important that our bodies get the right amounts to help sustain our life. It's always best to buy organic and local so the vitamins and minerals are at their optimum.

Low GI Food List: serving size one half cup TWICE a day.

1. Beans and legumes stabilize our blood sugar and are an amazing source of energy. Examples include: kidney, navy, black, cannellini, split peas, garbanzo and lentils. Be sure to only have one half-cup serving at lunch and one half cup with dinner along with a protein source and fiber (vegetable or fruit) source.
Black bean dip - one serving size (be sure to check serving size on bottle) for a snack or added to salad.

2. Squash winter squash, spaghetti squash, butternut and acorn

3. Yam or sweet potatoes (steamed, baked, broiled or roasted).

Whole Grains

If you are looking to lose weight or to see if you are sensitive to gluten, which is found in wheat, barley and rye or you might be sensitive to the Glyphosate that is in roundup ready wheat. You may want to consider withholding grains for 6-8 weeks or longer. By whole grains I mean 100% whole wheat, rye or barley. Look at the ingredients, that are listed; if you see whole-wheat flour, it means milled or refined and is processed. We want the ingredients to say 100% Whole Wheat.

I encourage no grains until you reach your weight loss goals but this is completely up to you. You will have greater weight loss success if you keep it out of your diet for 6-8 weeks. Even after two full weeks without whole grains you may begin to notice if you are sensitive or intolerant to the gluten found in wheat, barley or rye. When you add grains back into your diet and notice bloating, gas, diarrhea, constipation, and thickness around the middle, brain fog, headaches, and inflammation in joints or mood issues you may be sensitive to gluten. Journaling is helpful to keep track of potential symptoms. Symptoms could take 24-72 hours to show up. The best way to determine if you have an issue with gluten is to keep it out of your diet for 2-3 weeks and then document symptoms after reintroducing gluten products. If you think you have a problem, seek advice from a functional medicine physician to help guide you. If you can tolerate grains and you want to add them into your diet it's perfectly fine. Whole grains are high in fiber and very good for you. However, try to limit your grains to 1-3 servings per week not the 6-11 servings per day that the FDA recommends. I also would recommend Ezekiel products as they are fresh sprouted grains that digest more like a vegetable. You may find them in your grocery store in the freezer section. They have no preservatives so they will not last in your bread drawer for weeks like other bread. White pasta is not encouraged, wheat pasta if you are tolerating wheat but a better alternative is Quinoa Pasta and the Whole Grain Sprouted Quinoa. Pronounced (Keen-wah).

Spices

Add spices to your food as it adds flavor and spices have very healthy properties. Curry along with turmeric, cinnamon, and chilies are great spices to add to foods, as they are high in antioxidants and help regulate blood sugar levels and promote healthy circulation.

THINK PROTEIN & FIBER at EVERY MEAL while adding in a good fat.

It's important when eating this way to always be thinking about protein and fiber at every meal. Protein is necessary for weight loss. When eaten together with fiber it helps to burn calories and burn muscle. Eat 3-5 cups of (fiber) vegetables and a protein source at every meal (three times a day). Two times a day add a low Glycemic food from the GI list and twice a day eat healthy snacks of fresh fruits or veggies, with hummus or yogurt. You can use a minimal amount of essential fatty acids while trying to lose weight, just remember always portion control, read labels for serving sizes. Sounds simple right? Well, it is!

Here is an example of a typical day for 6-8 weeks:

BREAKFAST: An 8 ounce glass of warm lemon water
One protein source, 2-3 cups of veggies, and 1 low GI Example: One egg with peppers, onions and mushrooms sautéed with coconut oil with black bean dip, decaffeinated organic herbal tea or coffee

LUNCH: An 8 ounce glass of filtered water
One protein source and 2-3 cups of veggies
Example: A huge salad of dark leafy greens and veggies of your choice, with balsamic vinegar and a spray of extra virgin olive oil, add 4 ounces of chicken or tuna and a half a cup of low GI beans. One fruit serving

DINNER: **One protein source, 2-3 cups of veggies, and 1 low GI** Example: Same as above, a huge salad with balsamic vinegar and a spray of extra virgin olive oil with egg or chicken or tuna or tofu or shrimp or fish AND a low GI beans.

SNACKS: Many veggies or one fruit or small salad or one cup of soup or 9 almonds, cut up veggies with hummus, celery with 1-tablespoon nut-butter
Be creative, search for clean eating recipes, and be adventurous!

AFTER WEIGHT LOSS GOAL HAS BEEN REACHED

After 6-8 weeks OR when you have reached your weight loss goal (for some it may be 12-16 weeks or longer) you can begin adding good healthy grains back into your diet, for a breakfast change you may add some steel cut oats one half cup, with a few walnuts and low sugar fruit like berries, kiwi, pomegranate or green apples with one teaspoon of flax seed (freshly ground) and cinnamon. Google clean eating smoothies, there are many options on the web. One of my favorite smoothies is a handful of blueberries, one half cup of frozen banana, one half cup of unsweetened almond milk, as much spinach as my hand will hold and a teaspoon of ground flax or chia seeds. This is great for an on the go breakfast or anytime.

Lunch options after you've reached your weight loss goals may include 9 almonds or one portion of nuts or seeds of your choice added into your salad full of dark leafy greens and raw veggies, some beans or chickpeas, and possibly a cup of soup and a fresh fruit. The high fiber salad will balance the fructose in the fruit to keep your blood sugar stable. The same example is for dinner. You may add a protein source to each meal. Protein is necessary for weight loss. The rule of thumb is that when protein is eaten together with fiber it helps to burn calories and preserve muscle. So again, think protein and fiber at every meal and every snack.

Remember to keep journaling throughout this process until you have formed these new habits without giving food much thought. You are trading old habits with new ones and the research has shown that those who journal have a higher success rate than those who do not. Make sure you are planning for your week in advance, including your grocery shopping, and meal preparation. This is truly the key to success, as it will enable you to stay on track and avoid detours.

Restaurants

Choose restaurants that have healthier options, skip the bread, order water or Perrier w lemon, and ask how the protein or fish is prepared. Request food be steamed, broiled and without sauces. You can always order a double salad without cheese or croutons with a side of oil and vinegar and just ask for a double steamed vegetable as a side instead of a potato or rice.

Please keep in mind you are learning how to order healthier options not just for the next few weeks but for life.

What we choose to put into our mouths at home, parties or a restaurant will dictate our future health. If you adapt to this lifestyle, and you choose to eat good clean foods your can and will reduce the risk for disease. This amazing change will soon become a habit. Many clients find it isn't as difficult as they thought it would be and that they actually enjoy having better control over food choices. Remember, only YOU are responsible for what goes into your mouth.

There is no need to count points.

No need to weigh food.

There will be no counting of calories.

Chapter 4

Now it is Time to Move

For those of you involved in a structured exercise routine, keep it up. You will see greater results if you are already engaged in regular exercise of some sort AND when you combine exercise with this prescription of healthy eating. Both should be incorporated to keep you at optimal physical health.

Let me be clear, if exercising was as easy as calories in equal calories out everyone in the gym would be thin and you and I both know that it's not the case. You would have to walk about 3500 steps, for about a half hour just to burn off one piece of chocolate cake, and how many times have you seen someone working out with a Gatorade in his or her hands? Do you have any idea how much sugar is in one Gatorade? There are about 32 grams in a 20-ounce bottle. Truth is all the exercise in the world will not slim your hips if you are eating a poor diet. One of my clients was working out in a gym with a trainer 5 days a week for 4 years and was very discouraged that she couldn't lose any weight. She had gained muscle and improved her endurance over that time but couldn't shed a pound. She began this very same prescription to better health, combined her work out with eating good whole foods, and she is the now the size she was in high school at 42 years old. I cannot tell you how very pleased she is with her results and continues both eating well and exercising religiously.

Exercise AND eating well is extremely important for optimal health. The two work hand in hand to reduce belly fat, build muscle, strengthen your heart, decrease inflammation (the precursor to all disease), balance hormones, help with detoxification, improve brain function, and is great for your sex life! So there you have it: eating well and moving are critical to your prescription to good health.

Now if you are new to exercise, please consult your health care physician before beginning and don't do too much too soon. However, it is important to be thinking about what type of exercise you should be doing too. The research shows that to form a new habit you need to do it regularly. Creating a new habit takes three full weeks of doing something regularly that means every day! That doesn't mean you have to begin with a 45-minute aerobic workout right off the bat. Start slowly doing something you love, say for15 minutes then work up to 30 minutes. You will be more inclined to stick with something if you enjoy it. Then over a few weeks, work up to doing something every day for at least 40-45 minutes. What do you love to do, bike, hike, walk, kayak, yoga, or golf? Think about this for a minute because doing something you like will give you the motivation to do it daily. So pick something you enjoyed as a kid or mix it up so you are not bored. Get up and start moving every day even if you don't feel like it, do it anyway.

When you finish you will feel so much better mentally and physically. The messages you tell yourself determine your outcome so be positive and say to yourself, "I will and I can," then make an appointment with yourself and to get it done.

It's important to listen to your body; there is no one exercise that is perfect for everyone. You may need a vigorous aerobic exercise or weight lifting to help you feel more stable and gain strength or you may benefit from a gentler exercise to increase your flexibility and calm your mind.

There is no right or wrong time to get physical exercise. It is completely up to you. It's a good way to deal with stress and it helps the feel-good brain chemicals boost your mood. So whenever you can fit it into your schedule it will help you feel more energized. It's truly a matter of personal choice. Try to be cognizant of making it convenient and working at your own comfort level that way it will enhance your chances of doing it regularly.

Regular planned exercise is the best but remember it can take many forms. Parking far away from your destination, taking the stairs at work instead of the elevator, walking with your children or dog for 30 minutes is sometimes better for you than nothing. What do you think will get you moving? The biggest challenge is to find the exercise you enjoy and build it into your life on a regular basis. Everyone regardless of size or age should be incorporating movement into their daily life.

BMI (body mass index) we hear this mentioned all the time and since my specialty is not fitness I have a little different take on this number. BMI body mass index does not account for how much weight you have from muscle mass or body fat. I've often heard of athletes who had very high BMI because of muscle and not fat, similarly you can have a person who is "skinny fat" with a low BMI and very little muscle but fat inside. There is so much more to look at like weight, blood pressure, blood sugar levels, and cholesterol breakdown of LDL & HDL. There are thin people, who can be very sick, thin people can have illnesses and die of cancer, not just those who are overweight. So it's important to look at all the information and put all the pieces of the puzzle together that warrant keeping disease factors at bay. So while some health professionals use BMI is the primary measurement, I believe waist measurements is also a good indicator of a health risk. People of normal weight with big bellies are at a higher risk for death. A 2010 study published in "JAMA" Internal Medicine" cited that an increase in waist size was associated with a higher death rate regardless of BMI. So as you take your own measurements you may see if you fall into the high-risk category and you can work towards the goal of the current guidelines. To decrease your risk of disease and death, a woman's waist measurement should be below 35 inches and for men 40 or below. However, if you are less than 5 feet tall you should keep your waist measurement less than half your height. These guidelines are for the general public. Nevertheless, everyone should be eating healthy and exercising to decrease his or her risk for disease regardless of size.

STRESS... We all have it! It is part of our everyday life whether we like it not. Some stress is necessary but too much stress causes wear and tear emotionally, physically and mentally. There really isn't a magic formula for getting rid of stress in our lives but we can do some stress management by being proactive. Schedule and plan your time effectively with small breaks so you do not over commit all the time. I have learned over the years to say, "No" and not feel guilty. Try to not alleviate stressful symptoms with sugar and alcohol all that does is numb your thoughts temporarily. Balance is extremely important in life; I won't over commit myself just to be the perfect homemaker, wife, mother of three, grandmother, volunteer, pastoral care visitor, student, coach, and even an author. I have learned the hard way. Stress can cause disease; stress can negatively affect my autoimmune disease and probably contributed to my thyroid cancer. So, it's OK to say, "No" to some things to prevent taking on more than you can handle. Take some time out of your day to reflect on the things you are grateful for. There is so much negativity that surrounds us; we are so caught up in the day in and day out that we don't even notice that we are breathing. We should be grateful for every breath!

Just take a few minutes every now and again to stop and think about all that is going well in your life and while you are doing that, take in some slow deep breaths.

Yoga is a great way to meditate on all the good in your life. It is a great stress reliever.

Schedule regular massages.

Keep to an exercise routine.

Aim for 7-9 hours of sleep a night.

If you stick to this prescription combined with this good health eating plan, you will begin feeling good physically and mentally.

Journaling can also help reduce stress, try to be diligent about writing down your feelings good bad or indifferent. Getting those feelings out on paper helps you not only with self-reflection but self-exploration and helps with accountability and reduces our level of stress. Do not ever feel that you cannot ask for help. If you feel you need help in this area, please find someone that can help you. Chronic Stress can lead to many other health problems from heart disease, to depression and low self-esteem. I will address stress more in the last chapter. So if you aren't handling your stress well please seek out a professional.

Chapter 5

Eat Real Food
Not
Processed Food

Do you take the time to read labels? If you are anything like me, I believed everything manufacturers advertised on the front of their packaging. I have since learned otherwise; if you think advertisers tell the whole truth about what is in their food, think again! It's so important to look at the ingredients that are listed on the back of EVERY package and to question how safe that food actually is.

Did you know that the FDA (Food and Drug Administration) is supposed to determine the safety of our food? There are many different governmental agencies involved in regulating specific food, meat, drugs, toys, etc. The way I understand it is, when it comes to food additives (food like things) the FDA evaluates the additives in two ways: 1). Accepted daily intake (ADI) 2). Estimated Daily Intake (EDI). Simply put, if the EDI is less than the ADI, the ingredient can be considered safe. Since 1997 the research has been left up to the private companies who market their products with the additives NOT the FDA.

The companies inform the FDA of the substance, the intended use of that substance and the basis for granting their additives as GRAS (Generally regarded as safe). Then the FDA approves this based on their individual studies. This to me seems to be a conflict of interest and the FDA should do more independent studies over many years themselves before allowing them into our processed foods. Instead the opposite happens: they allow additives into the foods for many years and take the wait and see approach. It is now very apparent in my eyes that these additives have become highly suspect to contributing to the many diseases we have today. The system seems to be fundamentally broken and should be revisited. We have a broken health care system and many Americans who are ill from disease. It is my opinion that we might be better served if the FDA would do their own research and start with the food additives, GMO's, pesticides, herbicides and fungicides and get back to the food of yesterday. It's just might be very possible that many of our diseases would start to decline.

Trans-fat

When you look at the front of a package that says, "NO TRANS-FAT" what do you think? Usually that means there are no trans-fats in that package right? We all know trans-fats have been shown to cause coronary artery disease, so we aren't going to buy something with trans-fat in it right? What if you aren't looking at the ingredient label and you believe the front of the packaging? You would be seriously misled as the FDA has allowed companies to put as much as

0.5 g of trans-fatty acid in their products and list it as "ZERO trans-fat." It's extremely important to read the ingredient label to see if you see the words "Partially hydrogenated oil" as this means that you are in fact eating trans-fatty acid (TFA). Guess where else trans-fats are used every day that you may not be aware of? How about the oil that's in fryers at restaurants? From fast food restaurants to fine dining restaurants, many fry in trans-fats. It's important to inquire what type of grease they are frying your chicken fingers or Chicken Milanese in. The only way to know is to ask because if you don't that secret ingredient although it may taste good, over time may lead to cardiovascular disease!

Low Fat

Does low fat really mean low fat? Unfortunately, sugar has replaced the fat because it tastes good. You are better off eating the real deal, the full fat food item rather than low fat or light anything. If you look at the front of the product it might say "light" but how light is it? In looking at the sugar content it may be loaded with sugar and additionally have a list chemicals you can't even pronounce. Again, if you cannot pronounce an ingredient please do not eat it. Always look at the sugar content on the back of the package.

Natural Flavoring

Natural flavorings sound good don't they? I mean after all it is NATURAL right? Well, the truth is, it is impossible to know what Natural flavorings really are because they do not list them. It could be flavorings from anything that is approved by the FDA to be used in our food, and are not specified. Natural Flavorings sound appetizing and seem healthy right? Well, what if I told you "Natural Flavors" especially strawberry and vanilla come from the anal glands of a beaver. It's true! I'm sorry to say that as long as it's natural and comes from nature the FDA approves of it. Is it good for us? Well, there is no nutritional value in beaver glands so I'll let you be the judge of that.

Canola Oil

Have you heard that canola oil is one of the best oils to use? Many chefs, registered dietitians and many recipes call for and suggest we use canola oil as "the best" oil because it is rich in mono saturated fat with omegas III acids, which are also good for our health. Sorry to be the bearer of bad news BUT canola oil is a fake food! There is no canola "plant" that makes oil, like olives that when pressed make olive oil. Canola is a genetically modified rapeseed that was traditionally used in Asia but contains high levels of a toxic substance called Erucic acid. It is an artificially created oil that was derived from Canadian Oil, Low Acid thus we have (CANOLA) It started to be marketed in the United States in 1980 and the FDA approves is at "GRAS" (Generally

Regarded As Safe) in the United States. I don't know about you but that is not the oil I want to put in my body.

Food Dyes

Did you eat fruit loops as a child? How about bright orange cheese puffs? They are good right? Sure they taste good but did you know that food with food dyes have a warning label in Europe? The British government asked the manufacturers in their country to remove artificial colors from their food back in 2009. However, here in the USA these dyes are so common and are found in colored drinks, baked goods, Jell-o and even M&M candy. Dr. Mercola states these dyes are one of the most dangerous food additives linking them to cancers, organ damage, birth defects, allergies, hyper- activity and other behavioral problems in children. Even Dr. Feingold a pediatrician and allergist, a pioneer in his field, who developed a program in the1970's that eliminated artificial colorings, flavorings, artificial sweeteners, and preservatives like BHA and BHT (which are derived from crude oil gasoline). Many of his studies confirmed the dangers of these additives especially with children diagnosed with ADHD. Although much of his research was challenged he did help many through the "Feingold Program." All we have to do is take a look almost 50 years later and see all the children we have on ADHD medication. Instead of promoting such a diet for some, it would be better to pressure the FDA to demand that such toxic chemicals be removed from our food!

These dyes are listed in our food ingredients as "Yellow No.5," "Red 40," "Blue#1,"but don't be fooled as they are in our cosmetics and medicine too. Other non-desirable additives are MSG, sodium benzoate, nitrates (found in luncheon meats), and sulfites. Yes, I know these additives have been around for hundreds of years but years ago cotton candy and the yearly candy cane was a treat. Today we are consuming these dyes in many of our foods all day every day. In the 1940s kids had "white" toothpaste today it's multicolored. Just yesterday I heard that a toothpaste manufacturer announced that they would remove the tiny plastic micro beads from their toothpaste because they have been causing dental problems by getting stuck between the teeth. The micro beads are made from plastic, the same plastic they make grocery bags and bottles from, unfortunately they are not biodegradable, so how harmful is it if you swallow them? The FDA again approves their use as a food additive; it's NOT even a Food!

I used to eat Corn flakes when I was a child, that's before they were genetically modified. Remember ALL the corn today is genetically altered with round up unless you are buying non-GMO corn.

The food today is not like it was 20-30 years ago. Fruit loops and fruity pebbles are loaded with the artificial dyes. What did you eat on your pie during the holidays? I had real whipped cream on my desserts as a child; now we have this chemical called "cool whip" that everyone uses. Cool whip has hydrogenated vegetable oils, GMO high fructose corn syrup and natural and artificial flavorings among some other chemicals. It's unbelievable to me that these dangerous disease-causing additives are allowed. We really need to pay attention to the ingredients that can seriously do us harm in the long run. If no one else cares about our health and the health of our nation we need to.

I share these facts with you, so you will become more cognizant of what is in your food these days. You must become a label and ingredient reader. It is vitally important not to just believe what is on the front of every box, bag or carton. Google for yourself ingredients you are unfamiliar with to know if they are harmful to you or not. Do not rely on what the FDA regards as GRAS products that are in our food. Some foods are made exclusively in a manufacturing plant and are regarded as food when really they are "food like things" that have little to no nutritional value at all. Stick with the REAL food that comes from the ground, the REAL Plant food.

Very briefly I'd like to address the USDA (United States Department Agriculture) food pyramid recommendations. May I respectfully state, their food pyramid is outdated as they encourage 6-11 servings of grains a day. It's placed at the bottom of the pyramid making it one of the most foundational foods in your diet. It's no wonder we have a childhood diabetes problem with all those servings of breads, cereals, rice and pasta. It's like eating a bowl full of sugar every time you eat them, as they are "simple carbohydrates that turn into sugar."

Stick to this prescription to better health; lose the sugar and follow more of the Mediterranean diet to keep your body healthy. Yes, it is true! There are several things we cannot control in our world and we still may suffer from some diseases genetically or inherently, but we do not need to put ourselves at added risk especially when we educate ourselves about the real dangers of the relationship between food and disease. There is a strong correlation between Diet and Good Health and Diet and Disease. Only we can be responsible for what goes into our bodies. Just eat good whole foods from the earth as your prescription to better health. Folks, it's not rocket science. This plan is a no-starvation plan. Nutrient dense foods can be eaten anytime and should be eaten 90% of the time. They are less in calories so the more you eat the more you'll lose. The other 10% of foods are those that are still good for you but are higher in calories and fat like nuts, whole grains, fish and meat.

Alcohol

While trying to lose weight, the rule of thumb is no alcohol. Drinking may sabotage your weight loss goals. Alcohol has extra calories so it is not advised to skip a meal in place of an alcoholic beverage. It's best to eat first or include a work out on that day you plan to have a cocktail or two to help offset the extra calories. If you must consume an alcoholic drink, then my suggestion is to have a wine spritzer or a vodka and water or Tequila. A great alternative to wine would be Perrier water with lemon, club soda or seltzer water with lemon or lime. Hard liquor contains about 100 calories per shot so it's not good to add other ingredients or soda. All sweet drinks have sugar, thus more calories so be careful.

Chapter 6

You're Sweet Enough

Balancing the mind ~ the body ~ and the spirit ~ for wellness and healing

There are many ways to infuse balance into your life besides balancing nutrition and physical exercise. Don't get me wrong, good nutrition and physical exercise is absolutely necessary for optimal wellness and general health, so that covers the physical body, but equally important is the balancing of the mind and the spirit to balance life! By balancing your life putting all three together will make not only your life sweet but it will make you sweet enough! What I mean by this is, there are many reasons why we eat; I've already gone over the sugar, addiction part, now let's talk about emotions and stress, they play a big part in why some try to comfort themselves with food.

Mental Health

If you are dealing with mental health issues understand that food and mood go together. Stress is huge! Stress is a physical and emotional reaction. Everyone experiences stress and the reactions we have to stress can have positive or negative consequences.

A small amount of stress is helpful to allow us to deal with daily problems constructively to meet the challenges we are faced with daily. However, stress on a continual basis has very negative effects within our body and can cause heart disease, high blood pressure, and even depression. It is important to identify what causes stress in you in order to control it. Some situations are easier than others to identify. We need to take a look at ourselves and ask the questions: Do I have headaches, muscle tension, shaky hands, fatigue, insomnia, heartburn, am I nervous, confused, worried, irritable, and unable to concentrate? It's important to identify what is causing these symptoms.

Can you list 5 things below that may be causing you stress?
1.
2.
3.
4.
5.

Once you understand your stressors then you can take action and try to lesson them.

Ask yourself the following questions: Are you doing too many things at once?

If so then it's important to prioritize your tasks. Do one thing at a time.

Am I having a difficult time getting my point across?

Improve communication by listening, smiling, giving compliments and by expressing yourself assertively.

Do I share my thoughts with those I love?

Sharing thoughts with your spouse, your children a parent or friends is important, communicate your needs wants and desires effectively.

Do you feel stuck at work with a job you despise?

Don't be afraid to ask for advice. Sometimes others can see a way out or can help you with a better way to balance your workload or help refer you for a different job. Are you allowing time for self-care?

Make time for fun and relaxation.

How is your spirituality?

Are you finding time to appreciate all you have and all you are able to do?

Who comes along side you spiritually helping you with the strength and encouragement you need daily?

Possibly you should explore this further.

It's important to look at where you are dissatisfied in these areas and work on ways to bring them into a healthy balance. Does that make sense?

Take a good look at your relationships, are they strained? Are they causing you stress? How do you think you can you turn those relationships around to be less stressful in your life? Most often than not, it is how you react to that stressful relationship that will dictate internal healthy or unhealthy emotions. If it's a spouse and you've made the decision to stay, then have you thought about counseling? Even if the spouse will not go, you need to go for you!

It is important to work on skills and coping mechanisms to keep your stress levels balanced. Stress is something that we have not only with our spouses, families, and friends but also with our work associates, work responsibilities, possibly a lack of finances.

It's good to recognize what areas in your life are out of balance and then seek the appropriate means and take action to make them better. If there are real problems causing you stress, they will not go away. The problems just get worse in time if you are not actively working on making them better balanced. It's important to recognize your stressors and if you cannot find ways to reduce your stress and need help finding strategies that will work seek out a qualified councilor to help because the stress will get worse over time. There is good information and a stress quiz at www.helpguide.org

It's equally important not to hold onto the things that cause us a great deal of pain and suffering. This is something you can do right now starting today? Give up on the things that no longer serve you well.

Are You Sweet Enough?

Now is the time when I ask **Do YOU want to BE SWEET** enough? You can be if you follow some very simple guidelines:

"Love yourself. Forgive yourself. Be true to yourself. How you treat yourself sets the standard for how others will treat you." ~By Steve Maraboli

Learn how to Love your Sweet Self!

1.) Give up the need to always be right. Who cares? **JUST BE SWEET!**

2.) Give up the need for control. Allow others to be who they are and accept them just as they are. **JUST BE SWEET AND DO NOT WORRY ABOUT THEM.**

3.) Take responsibility for your own life. Don't blame others for what you have or do NOT have or how your feeling or do NOT feel. **Own it SWEETLY.**

4.) Stop the negative talk. Believe in yourself. Recognize your inner beauty. **YOU are Sweet Enough!** Do NOT believe everything your mind is telling you. Always ask yourself if it is true. Then change that negative thought to a positive one. Positive approaches help to manage all stress **~ ALLOWS YOU TO BE JUST A LITTLE SWEETER!**

5.) Give up the need to impress others. **YOU ARE SWEET ENOUGH!**

6.) Embrace change. Change will help you improve your life. Seek out better ways to handle and react to others as well as keeping growth and learning alive daily in your life regardless of your age! Now that's **SWEET!**

7.) STOP complaining. **BE SWEET**~ No one likes to hear from a complainer and no one can make you unhappy, sad, or depressed. It's how YOU view a situation and how you view your own response. Respond in kind and with positivity always.

8.) Give up your fears; fear is all in the mind it is something created just by you.
Let go of the past, and look forward to the **SWEET** future.

9.) Be present in all you do, set boundaries, set goals, stay focused, be courageous, forgive yourself and others so you can enjoy an abundant life: it is much too short!

10.) **LOVE yourself ~ because YOU are worth it ~ YOU ARE SWEET ENOUGH!**
These helpful hints are indeed a prescription to keep you nutritionally, physically, mentally, and spiritually **SWEET ENOUGH!**

You do not need all that sugar!

My goal in writing this book is to help you be the BEST you can BE. Losing the sugar from your diet by following my prescription for better health is going to help you keep diseases at bay or possibly help reverse disease if you already have it. We have a major health care crisis on our hands with diabetes and obesity. Much of that has to do with our daily intake of sugar. It's not just the elderly either; children are getting type II Diabetes for the first time in 30 years. As a Health Care Professional (R.N) and Holistic Health Coach I am extremely concerned about the future of our children and the people of today. It is my hope and dream to make a difference, one person at a time creating a ripple effect that could possibly change the world. I commend each and every one of you reading this book because it means you care enough about yourself to try to make better changes in your nutrition to be a healthier YOU! Thank you for letting me into your lives. If it weren't for your desire to take control over your own health, this book wouldn't have been written. Hippocrates said, "Let Food Be Thy Medicine." It is still true today.

It is my hope that this prescription to better health encourages you to change your lifestyle, eat healthier, exercise more, reduce stress, sleep better, and take better care of your mind, body and spirit for wellness and healing. So let's "Lose the Sugar" folks "You Are Sweet Enough."

Be Well My Friends,

Coach Karen Marie

Chapter 7

Juicing and Smoothies

To get in a good portion of your vitamins in a drink, you may want to try juicing or a smoothie. It is a quick and easy way to obtain your vitamins and nutrients. I consume both for extra energy; a smoothie can be used in the morning as a meal replacement or you can juice as a snack. Smoothies contain more fruit AND fiber while juicing is loaded with dark leafy greens and vegetables and has the fiber removed.

Juicing ~ **Removes the fiber**!

Wash all veggies and fruits first ~ Organics are preferred ~ Fresh juice optimally should be consumed right after making it and on an empty stomach so the vitamins and minerals get right into the bloodstream. I have made the juice in an airtight container the night before when I have had early morning activities, but remember, the fresher the better. Juicing REMOVES the fiber and can also be used if you need to be on bowel rest for some reason, example diverticulitis. I like to use juice as a snack in the afternoon. Green juice helps me feel more energized in afternoon. A rule of thumb is to wait 20 minutes after drinking juice to consume a meal or wait 2 hours after a meal to consume a juice. Juicing reduces the amount of energy your body uses for digestion but gives you the boost of extra vitamins and minerals in one glass. Juicing should be used as a snack not a meal replacement. It's good to juice the vegetables and fruits you may NOT want to eat.

Rinse your juicer immediately after using to save time or it will be hard to clean. Here is a suggestion for juicing but you can Google many recipes.

Pick ONE for the base: one half of a bunch of celery or 2 cucumbers

Then add ONE leafy green (a handful) make sure you use a variety: spinach, kale, Swiss chard, mustard greens, collards, dandelions, and arugula.

Then add ONE Fruit: apple, (grapefruit, lime, lemon, peels removed), pears, and berries.

Then add ONE optional: ginger, broccoli stems, cayenne pepper, parsley, cilantro or mint.

Smoothie ~ **Contains the fiber!**

This is a favorite of mine. It is simple and easy and sometimes I'll make it the night before and just re-blend it in the morning with some ice. Smoothies CONTAIN the fiber and can be used in place of a meal. Smoothies should be consumed within 12 hours just make sure it is in an airtight container in the refrigerator.

> One small container of unsweetened plain organic yogurt
> One-fourth cup unsweetened almond milk
> A handful of blueberries, strawberries, blackberries, or raspberries.
> A handful of spinach
> 1 teaspoon of chia seeds

I add chia seeds because they help with satiety and are great for drawing toxins out of the body. (When made the night before, chia seeds swell and turn into a gel.)
You can also add any "superfoods" to your smoothies. Some examples of superfoods are coconut oil, chia seeds, flax seeds, goji berries, spirulina, cacao powder, cacao nibs, avocado, and hemp protein. Each superfood has their own set of nutrients. It's important to research what you would like to add and why. By bringing superfoods into your smoothies will

enhance the flavor and your nutrition so pick them appropriately to enhance your health.

Karen Calandra has received Holistic training at the Institute of Integrated Nutrition in New York City. She offers workshops, public speaking and individual and group sessions to support her clients in making healthy and positive changes to ensure success to live an inspired and fulfilling life.

For more information visit:
www.karencalandrahealthcoach.com

Chapter 8

Testimonials

"Phase one of my journey was losing 46 pound in 11 weeks. I've made the commitment to eat right and stick this out to get healthier! I don't count calories or measure my food. This is the way I could eat for a lifetime. I feel dramatically better physically and emotionally. I owe a great deal of thanks to Coach Karen and her constant support and encouragement throughout the process."

M.P. (47 years old)

"My doctor was so excited about my weight loss, she said I am the gold star of the day. My cholesterol went from 176 to 133 and my triglycerides went from 165 to 56. I bought my first pair of size 6 jeans after losing 32 pounds. I am so excited! I know I can do this for life! Thank you, Coach Karen for helping me believe in myself and equipping me with the tools to change my eating habits for life!"

K.G. (56 years old)

"I am ecstatic that I participated in Coach Karen's Prescription to Better Health Program. I am convinced that this is my new eating style for life! I have experienced a great deal of success during and after the program. Not only did I lose 25 pounds, but here is the BEST news of all. My recent visit with my cardiologist allowed us to analyze my blood work before and after my new style of eating. Your program played more of a significant effect on my risk factors for heart attack and stroke than all the medicine I have been taking for three years after my heart attack. Before this lifestyle change my overall cholesterol was 180, triglycerides 212 and my LDL was 97. After changing my eating habits, thanks to you, my cholesterol was 108, triglycerides 97 and my LDL was 45. I cannot thank you enough for all your help and this amazing program. My results were more than amazing and I am so glad I have learned to eat this and not that; it just may save my life!

M.C. (63 years old)

"If you are getting serious about improving your health and looking & feeling better check this out! I just graduated last night from the Prescription to Better Health Program with Coach Karen Marie, and I've never felt better (not even in my 20's). I am back in my "skinny" jeans and my hair and skin look great and IT'S EASY! This is not some fad diet it is a way of eating well for the rest of your life. No pills, crazy cleanses, just eating fresh, wholesome REAL foods and skipping the sugars and processed JUNK that do NOTHING good for our bodies. If you want to ward off disease, look and feel better JUST DO IT! My health Coach Karen Marie was supportive, motivating, encouraging and really wants people to feel better and be healthy! What do you have to lose? Maybe some pounds and inches! What do you have to gain? Definitely a healthier lifestyle, more years with your family, and control over your life.

S.L. (44 years old)

"This way of life works, it's just that simple. I've yo-yoed with my weight ever since my first series of diets began in high school. I've restricted, I've counted calories, I've drank and eaten prepackaged meals. I'd lose weight, go back to my old habits, gain it back, start a new diet and repeat. When I learned about this prescription to better health and heard about all the success others were having, I signed up purely for the goal of losing weight to look good. Something clicked for me at Coach Karen Marie's free introductory seminar; a light switch was turned on and suddenly health and wellness jumped ahead of just looking thin or fitting into those skinny jeans in the back of my closet. I never thought I'd make it through the detox week but have since done mini detoxes with ease. By eating the right foods, I've never gone hungry or felt deprived a side effect of most crash diets. I've been able to come off almost all my allergy medication and pain medication for a chronic bad back. My body is smaller, more tone and healthy too! My mood and general outlook have improved and I no longer get the 3 o'clock slump at my desk. I do NOT crave sugar like I used to and I really feel as though I am over my sugar addiction. Like I said, this way of life (it's not a diet) works … it's just that simple."

R.F. (42 years old)

"Really enjoyed my experience with Coach Karen Marie. This program truly improved my overall health. I just had my doctor's appointment and had great lab reports: cholesterol 189, triglycerides 94, and blood glucose 86. I've lost weight and went down 3 pant sizes, my blood pressure has gone down significantly, such that my medical doctor stopped my blood pressure medication that I have been taking for the last 14 years. This Prescription to Better Health is a great program, easy to follow and a lifestyle I will continue to enjoy, Thank You Coach Karen Marie for equipping me with the tools that will last me a lifetime of Healthy Eating."

J.W. (64 years old)

Resources

The Department Of Health and Human Services
www.edc.gov/healthyyouth/obesity/facts.htm

www.cdc.gov/needphp/publications/factsheet/prevention/
pdf/obesity.pdf

Dr. Mark Hyman
www.nydailynews.com/life-style/health/dr-mark-hyman-
shows-deadly-sugar-addiction-article-1.1608553

Dirty Dozen list
www.ewg.org/foodnews/

GMO products
www.responsibletechnology.org/10-reasons-to-avoid-GMO

GMO labeling bills
Bigstory.ap.org/article/genetically-modified-foods-confuse-
consumers

2013 French research team
www.nature.com/news/study-linking-gm-maize-to-rat-
tumours-is-retracted-1.142 68

Mediterranean Diet Pyramid
www.oldwayspt.org

http://worldobserveronline.com/2012/04/25/15-things-you-should-give-up-to-be-happy

Portal.nysed.gov/portal/page/pref/CNKC/Nutrition_Page_pp/TransFatFactSheet.pdf

Articles.mercola.com/sites/articles/archive/2011/02/24/are-you-or-your-family-eating-toxic-food-dyes.aspx

TLS
Serenity is 1

Detox kit TLS

CPSIA information can be obtained at www.ICGtesting.com
Printed in the USA
LVOW10s0224150915

454106LV00031B/1894/P